Juicing Health

Dr. Monique Rodgers

Restored

Dr. Monique Rodgers

United States of America

Published by Shooting Stars Publishing House 2024

ISBN:

Dedication

To everyone who longs to have better health.

-Dr. Monique

Contents

Introduction

In a world where health trends come and go, juicing stands out as a timeless practice with profound benefits. By harnessing the pure, concentrated nutrients found in fresh fruits and vegetables, juicing offers a powerful way to nourish the body, boost energy levels, and promote overall well-being.

The benefits of juicing are numerous. From enhancing digestion to supporting detoxification, juicing delivers essential vitamins, minerals, and enzymes directly to your system, making it easier for your body to absorb and utilize these nutrients. It's a simple yet effective way to ensure you're getting the most out of what nature has to offer.

My journey into juicing began as a quest for better health and vitality. Like many, I found myself overwhelmed by the complexities of maintaining a balanced diet in a busy world. Juicing became a practical solution, allowing me to fuel my body with the nutrients it craved without the hassle of complicated meal preparations. As I delved deeper into the world of juicing, I discovered its transformative potential—not just for physical health, but for mental clarity and emotional well-being as well.

In this book, I invite you to explore the power of juicing with me. Whether you're a seasoned juicer or just beginning your journey, this guide will provide you with the knowledge, tools, and inspiration you need to make juicing an integral part of your life. Together, we'll unlock the secrets to better health, one glass of fresh juice at a time.

Chapter One

Understanding Juicing

Juicing has become a popular health practice for many people seeking a convenient way to boost their nutrient intake and improve their overall well-being. This chapter will explore the fundamentals of juicing, how it differs from blending, and the nutritional benefits that make it such a powerful addition to any health regimen.

What is Juicing?

Definition and Basics

At its core, juicing is the process of extracting the liquid from fresh fruits and vegetables, leaving behind the fibrous pulp. This liquid, known as juice, contains most of the vitamins, minerals, and phytonutrients present in the whole produce. The idea behind juicing is to concentrate these nutrients into a single, easy-to-consume beverage, allowing your body to absorb them more efficiently.

Juicing can be done using various types of juicers, including centrifugal, masticating, and twin-gear juicers. Each type of juicer works slightly differently, but the basic principle remains the same: to separate the juice from the solid parts of the fruit or vegetable. Centrifugal juicers, for example, use a spinning blade to shred the produce and a strainer to separate the juice from the pulp. Masticating juicers, on the other hand, crush the produce using a slow, grinding action, which is believed to preserve more nutrients due to the lack of heat generated during the process.

Difference Between Juicing and Blending

One common question that arises when discussing juicing is how it differs from blending. While both juicing and blending involve processing fruits and vegetables into a liquid form, the end results are quite different.

Blending, as the name suggests, involves combining whole fruits and vegetables in a blender, including the fiber, into a thick, smoothie-like consistency. This method retains all the fiber, which is essential for digestive health and helps to slow the absorption of sugar into the bloodstream.

Juicing, by contrast, removes the fiber, resulting in a more concentrated source of nutrients in a liquid form. This lack of fiber means that the nutrients in juice are absorbed more quickly by the body, providing an almost immediate boost of vitamins, minerals, and other beneficial compounds. However, because juice lacks fiber, it is important to consume it mindfully, particularly if the juice is high in natural sugars, such as those found in fruits like apples or oranges.

Both juicing and blending have their place in a balanced diet. Blending is ideal for those who want to increase their fiber intake and create more filling, meal-like beverages. Juicing is perfect for those looking to maximize their nutrient intake in a quick and easily digestible form. Many people find that incorporating both methods into their routine allows them to enjoy the best of both worlds.

Nutritional Benefits

Vitamins, Minerals, and Enzymes

One of the primary reasons people turn to juicing is to increase their intake of essential vitamins, minerals, and enzymes. Fresh fruits and vegetables are packed with these nutrients, which play crucial roles in maintaining health and preventing disease.

Vitamins such as vitamin C, vitamin A, and a range of B vitamins are abundant in fresh produce. These vitamins are essential for a variety of bodily functions, including immune system support, skin health, and energy production. Minerals like potassium, calcium, and magnesium are also plentiful in many fruits and vegetables, supporting bone health, muscle function, and cardiovascular health.

In addition to vitamins and minerals, fresh produce contains enzymes, which are biological catalysts that facilitate chemical reactions in the body. Enzymes are particularly important for digestion, helping to break down food into its component nutrients so that they can be absorbed and utilized by the body. Juicing helps to preserve these enzymes, especially when using cold-press or masticating juicers that generate less heat during the extraction process.

How Juicing Aids in Nutrient Absorption

One of the key advantages of juicing is its ability to enhance nutrient absorption. When you consume whole fruits and vegetables, the fiber in these foods slows down the digestive process, which is beneficial for managing blood sugar levels and promoting satiety. However, this can also mean that the absorption of certain nutrients is delayed.

Juicing, by removing the fiber, allows the body to absorb nutrients more rapidly. This can be particularly beneficial when you need a quick energy boost or when you're looking to flood your body with nutrients to support recovery from illness or intense physical activity. The rapid absorption of nutrients from juice can provide an immediate sense of vitality and well-being, making it an excellent option for starting your day or replenishing after a workout.

Moreover, the concentration of nutrients in juice means that you're getting a higher dose of vitamins, minerals, and phytonutrients in each glass. For example, it might take several servings of whole vegetables to match the nutrient content of a single glass of green juice. This concentration allows you to consume a variety of nutrients without having to eat large quantities of food, which can be particularly helpful for those with reduced appetites or specific dietary needs.

However, it's important to note that while juicing offers numerous benefits, it should not replace the consumption of whole fruits and vegetables. The fiber found in whole foods plays a critical role in maintaining digestive health, stabilizing blood sugar levels, and supporting heart health. Therefore, juicing should be seen as a complement to a balanced diet, rather than a substitute for whole foods.

This chapter provides a foundation for understanding what juicing is, how it differs from blending, and the nutritional benefits it offers. As you continue reading, you'll discover how to make the most of your juicing experience, from selecting the best ingredients to creating delicious, health-boosting recipes tailored to your specific needs. Whether you're new to juicing or looking to deepen your knowledge, this book will guide you on a journey toward better health, one glass of juice at a time.

Chapter Two

Getting Started with Juicing

Embarking on a juicing journey can be an exciting and transformative experience, but it's essential to start with the right tools and knowledge to maximize the benefits. In this chapter, we'll explore the different types of juicers available, discuss their pros and cons, and highlight the essential tools and equipment you'll need to make juicing an enjoyable and sustainable habit.

Choosing the Right Juicer

Types of Juicers

The first step in getting started with juicing is selecting the right juicer. There are three main types of juicers: centrifugal, masticating, and twin gear. Each type operates differently, and understanding these differences will help you choose the best option for your needs.

1. Centrifugal Juicers: These are the most common and widely available juicers on the market. Centrifugal juicers work by using a fast-spinning blade to shred the produce, while the centrifugal force separates the juice from the pulp. The juice is then collected in a separate container, ready to be enjoyed.

- Pros:

  - Speed: Centrifugal juicers are fast, making them a good choice for those who need a quick juice fix.

  - Availability: These juicers are widely available and come in a range of prices, making them accessible to most people.

  - Ease of Use: Centrifugal juicers are generally easy to use, making them ideal for beginners.

- Cons:

  - Heat: The high-speed spinning of the blade generates heat, which can destroy some of the enzymes and nutrients in the juice.

- Oxidation: The fast processing can introduce more air into the juice, leading to quicker oxidation and a shorter shelf life.

- Noise: Centrifugal juicers tend to be noisy, which might be a consideration for those juicing in the early morning or late at night.

2. Masticating Juicers (Slow Juicers): Also known as cold-press juicers, masticating juicers operate at a slower speed, using an auger to crush and press the produce to extract juice. This method is gentler on the produce and preserves more nutrients.

- Pros:

  - Nutrient Preservation: The slow, cold-press method helps preserve the enzymes, vitamins, and minerals in the juice.

  - Juice Yield: Masticating juicers typically extract more juice from the same amount of produce, making them more efficient.

  - Versatility: These juicers can handle a wider range of produce, including leafy greens, wheatgrass, and even nuts for making nut milk.

- Cons:

  - Speed: Masticating juicers are slower than centrifugal juicers, which might be a downside if you're in a hurry.

  - Price: These juicers tend to be more expensive due to their advanced technology and higher juice yield.

  - Cleaning: Masticating juicers often have more parts, which can make them a bit more cumbersome to clean.

3. Twin Gear Juicers (Triturating Juicers): Twin gear juicers use two interlocking gears to crush and grind the produce, extracting juice with minimal oxidation and maximum nutrient retention. These juicers are known for their efficiency and ability to handle a wide variety of produce.

- Pros:

  - Superior Juice Quality: Twin gear juicers produce juice with minimal oxidation, resulting in a longer shelf life and better nutrient retention.

- High Juice Yield: These juicers extract the maximum amount of juice from produce, making them highly efficient.

- Versatility: Like masticating juicers, twin gear juicers can handle a wide range of produce, including leafy greens and hard vegetables.

- Cons:

- Price: Twin gear juicers are the most expensive type of juicer, which may be a significant investment for some.

- Complexity: These juicers have more parts and require more time to clean, which might be a drawback for those seeking convenience.

- Size and Weight: Twin gear juicers are often larger and heavier, requiring more counter space and effort to move.

When choosing a juicer, it's important to consider your specific needs, budget, and how you plan to use the juicer. If you're new to juicing and want something quick and easy, a centrifugal juicer might be a good start. However, if you're serious about juicing and want to maximize the nutritional benefits, investing in a masticating or twin gear juicer could be worthwhile.

Essential Juicing Tools and Equipment

Must-Have Kitchen Tools for Juicing

Beyond the juicer itself, there are a few essential tools and equipment that can enhance your juicing experience and make the process smoother.

1. Cutting Board and Knife: A good-quality cutting board and a sharp knife are essential for prepping your produce. Invest in a sturdy cutting board that provides enough space to work comfortably and a

sharp knife that makes slicing through tough vegetables and fruits easier.

2. Strainer or Sieve: If you prefer your juice without any pulp, a fine mesh strainer or sieve can help remove any remaining solids from the juice, resulting in a smoother texture.

3. Juice Storage Containers: To store your juice, you'll need airtight containers, preferably made of glass, to preserve the freshness and prevent oxidation. Mason jars are a popular choice, as they are affordable, durable, and come in various sizes.

4. Citrus Juicer: If you plan on juicing citrus fruits frequently, a handheld citrus juicer or reamer can make the process faster and more efficient, ensuring you extract every last drop of juice.

5. Vegetable Peeler: Some fruits and vegetables may need to be peeled before juicing, especially if they're not organic. A good-quality vegetable peeler can make this task easier and quicker.

Tips for Maintaining and Cleaning Your Juicer

Proper maintenance and cleaning of your juicer are crucial for ensuring its longevity and maintaining the quality of your juice. Here are some tips to keep your juicer in top condition:

1. Clean Immediately After Use: Cleaning your juicer immediately after use prevents the pulp and juice residue from drying and sticking to the parts, making it easier to clean. Most juicers come with a cleaning brush to help remove debris from hard-to-reach areas.

2. Disassemble and Soak: Disassemble the juicer parts and soak them in warm, soapy water to loosen any remaining pulp and juice residue. This will make it easier to scrub away any stubborn bits.

3. Use a Cleaning Brush: A small cleaning brush, often provided with the juicer, is useful for scrubbing the fine mesh strainer or filter basket, where pulp can get trapped.

4. Avoid Harsh Chemicals: Use mild dish soap and warm water for cleaning. Avoid harsh chemicals that could damage the juicer's components.

5. Dry Thoroughly: After cleaning, make sure all the parts are completely dry before reassembling the juicer. This helps prevent mold and bacterial growth.

6. Regular Maintenance: Check your juicer's manual for any specific maintenance instructions, such as lubricating moving parts or

replacing filters. Regular maintenance will ensure your juicer runs smoothly and efficiently.

7. Store Properly: When not in use, store your juicer in a clean, dry place. If you use your juicer frequently, keeping it on the countertop can be convenient, but ensure it's covered to protect it from dust.

By choosing the right juicer and equipping yourself with the essential tools, you're setting yourself up for a successful juicing journey. With proper care and maintenance, your juicer will be a reliable companion in your quest for better health, providing you with fresh, nutrient-rich juices for years to come.

This chapter has provided you with the foundational knowledge to choose the right juicer and gather the essential tools needed for juicing. As you continue on this journey, remember that the key to successful juicing is not just the equipment, but also the joy and creativity you bring to the process. In the next chapter, we'll dive into selecting the best ingredients for your juices, ensuring that every glass you make is as nutritious and delicious as possible.

Chapter Three

Selecting Ingredients

The heart of any juice lies in its ingredients. The quality, freshness, and variety of fruits, vegetables, and superfoods you choose can make a significant difference in the nutritional value and taste of your juice. In this chapter, we'll explore the best fruits and vegetables for juicing, discuss the importance of selecting seasonal produce, and dive into the world of superfoods and add-ins that can elevate your juicing experience to a whole new level.

Fruits and Vegetables

Best Fruits and Vegetables for Juicing

When it comes to juicing, not all fruits and vegetables are created equal. Some are naturally more juice-friendly, yielding a higher volume of liquid, while others offer unique flavors and nutritional benefits. Below is a list of some of the best fruits and vegetables for juicing:

1. Apples: Apples are a juicing staple due to their high water content, natural sweetness, and pleasant flavor. They're also rich in vitamins, particularly vitamin C, and antioxidants that help protect the body against oxidative stress.

2. Carrots: Carrots are another popular juicing ingredient, known for their vibrant orange color and slightly sweet taste. They're packed

with beta-carotene, which the body converts into vitamin A, essential for healthy skin, vision, and immune function.

3. Celery: Celery is a hydrating vegetable with a high water content, making it perfect for juicing. It's also known for its anti-inflammatory properties and is a good source of potassium, which helps regulate blood pressure.

4. Cucumbers: Cucumbers are incredibly refreshing and hydrating, thanks to their high water content. They add a mild, crisp flavor to juices and are rich in vitamins K and C, as well as various antioxidants.

5. Spinach: Spinach is a nutrient-dense leafy green that's easy to juice and pairs well with both fruits and vegetables. It's a great source of iron, calcium, and vitamins A, C, and K, making it an excellent choice for boosting your juice's nutritional value.

6. Kale: Kale is another leafy green powerhouse, loaded with vitamins A, C, and K, as well as antioxidants and anti-inflammatory compounds. It has a slightly bitter taste, so it's often balanced with sweeter fruits like apples or oranges in juices.

7. Oranges: Oranges are a juicy and flavorful fruit that adds a burst of vitamin C to any juice. Their natural sweetness makes them a great base for many juice recipes, especially those featuring more bitter or earthy vegetables.

8. Beets: Beets have a deep, earthy flavor and a striking red color that adds vibrancy to any juice. They're rich in folate, manganese, and dietary nitrates, which can help improve blood flow and lower blood pressure.

9. Ginger: Although not a fruit or vegetable in the traditional sense, ginger is a fantastic add-in for juices. It has a spicy kick and offers numerous health benefits, including anti-inflammatory and digestive properties.

10. Pineapple: Pineapple is a tropical fruit that adds a sweet and tangy flavor to juices. It's also a good source of vitamin C and bromelain, an enzyme that aids digestion and has anti-inflammatory effects.

Seasonal Produce Guide

Using seasonal produce in your juicing routine not only ensures that you're getting the freshest and most flavorful ingredients but also supports local agriculture and can be more cost-effective. Here's a brief guide to help you choose the best seasonal produce for juicing throughout the year:

1. Spring: As winter fades, spring brings a variety of fresh, crisp produce ideal for juicing. Look for ingredients like strawberries, spinach, kale, carrots, and citrus fruits like oranges and lemons. Spring is also a great time for herbs like mint and parsley, which can add a refreshing twist to your juices.

2. Summer: Summer is the season of abundance, with a wide range of juicy, hydrating fruits and vegetables available. Cucumbers, watermelons, tomatoes, berries, peaches, and leafy greens are all in their prime. These ingredients are perfect for creating light, refreshing juices that help keep you cool and hydrated in the heat.

3. Fall: As the weather cools, fall brings heartier produce with deep, earthy flavors. Apples, pears, beets, carrots, and sweet potatoes are all excellent choices for juicing in the fall. This is also the time to start incorporating more root vegetables and spices like ginger and cinnamon into your juices for a warming effect.

4. Winter: Winter may seem like a challenging time for fresh produce, but there are still plenty of nutrient-rich options available.

Citrus fruits like oranges, grapefruits, and lemons are at their peak, offering a much-needed vitamin C boost. You can also juice winter greens like kale and Swiss chard, as well as root vegetables like carrots and beets, to create nourishing, immune-boosting juices.

By selecting seasonal produce, you can ensure that your juices are not only delicious and nutritious but also aligned with nature's cycles. This approach allows you to enjoy a wide variety of flavors and nutrients throughout the year.

Superfoods and Add-ins

Benefits of Adding Superfoods

Superfoods are nutrient-dense ingredients that can provide an extra boost to your juices, enhancing their health benefits and nutritional value. These foods are often rich in antioxidants, vitamins, minerals, and other compounds that support overall health and well-being. Adding superfoods to your juices can help:

1. Boost Immunity: Many superfoods are rich in antioxidants and vitamins that strengthen the immune system, helping the body fight off infections and illnesses.

2. Enhance Energy Levels: Superfoods like spirulina and chlorella are packed with essential nutrients that can help increase energy levels and improve physical performance.

3. Improve Digestion: Ingredients like chia seeds and flaxseeds are high in fiber, which aids digestion and promotes a healthy gut.

4. Support Detoxification: Superfoods such as wheatgrass and turmeric contain compounds that support the body's natural detoxification processes, helping to eliminate toxins and promote liver health.

5. Promote Skin Health: Many superfoods, like acai berries and goji berries, are rich in antioxidants that protect the skin from damage and promote a healthy, glowing complexion.

Common Superfoods and Their Health Benefits

Here are some common superfoods that you can easily incorporate into your juicing routinc:

1. Spirulina: Spirulina is a blue-green algae that's incredibly rich in protein, vitamins, minerals, and antioxidants. It's known for its ability to boost energy, support detoxification, and improve overall health. A small amount of spirulina powder can be added to your juices for a nutrient boost.

2. Chia Seeds: Chia seeds are tiny seeds that pack a big nutritional punch. They're high in omega-3 fatty acids, fiber, and protein. When added to juices, they help improve digestion and keep you feeling full longer.

3. Turmeric: Turmeric is a bright yellow spice known for its powerful anti-inflammatory and antioxidant properties. Adding a small piece of fresh turmeric root or a pinch of turmeric powder to your juice can help reduce inflammation and support joint health.

4. Ginger: Ginger is another potent anti-inflammatory and digestive aid. It adds a spicy kick to juices and can help soothe the digestive system, reduce nausea, and support immune health.

5. Flaxseeds: Flaxseeds are rich in omega-3 fatty acids, fiber, and lignans, which have antioxidant properties. Adding ground flaxseeds to your juices can help improve digestion and support heart health.

6. Wheatgrass: Wheatgrass is a young grass of the wheat plant and is packed with chlorophyll, vitamins, minerals, and amino acids. It's known for its detoxifying properties and ability to boost energy levels and support overall health.

7. Acai Berries: Acai berries are small, dark purple berries that are high in antioxidants, particularly anthocyanins. They help protect the body from oxidative stress and support heart health. Acai powder can be added to juices for a fruity, nutritious boost.

8. Goji Berries: Goji berries are bright red berries that are rich in antioxidants, vitamins, and minerals. They're known for their ability to support immune function, improve skin health, and promote longevity. Goji berry powder or juice can be easily incorporated into your recipes.

By incorporating superfoods and nutrient-rich add-ins into your juices, you can create powerful, health-boosting beverages that go beyond basic nutrition. These ingredients not only enhance the flavor and variety of your juices but also provide targeted health benefits that support your overall well-being.

As you explore the world of juicing, selecting the right ingredients is key to maximizing the health benefits and enjoyment of your juices.

Whether you're focusing on seasonal produce, adding nutrient-dense superfoods, or simply experimenting with new flavors, the choices you make can have a profound impact on your health and vitality. In the next chapter, we'll discuss how to create balanced, delicious juice recipes that cater to your specific health goals and taste preferences.

Chapter Four

Juicing Recipes for Health Goals

Juicing isn't just a delicious way to enjoy fruits and vegetables; it can also be a powerful tool for achieving specific health goals. Whether you're looking to increase your energy levels, detoxify your body, support weight loss, or boost your immune system, there's a juice recipe that can help. In this chapter, we'll explore various juice recipes tailored to these health goals, along with the benefits of specific ingredients that promote vitality, detoxification, weight management, and immune health.

Energy and Vitality

Recipes to Boost Energy

When you're feeling sluggish or fatigued, the right combination of fruits and vegetables can provide a natural energy boost. Juices rich in vitamins, minerals, and antioxidants can help fuel your body and mind, giving you the vitality you need to power through your day. Here are some energy-boosting juice recipes:

1. Morning Energizer

- Ingredients: 2 apples, 2 carrots, 1 orange, 1-inch piece of ginger

- Instructions: Juice all the ingredients together. The apples and carrots provide natural sugars and fiber, while the orange adds a burst of vitamin C. Ginger helps to stimulate circulation and metabolism, giving you a gentle boost of energy.

2. Green Power Juice

- Ingredients: 1 cucumber, 2 celery stalks, 1 handful of spinach, 1 apple, 1 lemon

- Instructions: Juice all the ingredients together. This juice is packed with chlorophyll from the spinach and cucumber, which helps oxygenate your blood and increase energy levels. The lemon adds a refreshing tang and helps to alkalize the body.

3. Beetroot Bliss

-Ingredients: 1 beetroot, 2 carrots, 1 apple, 1-inch piece of turmeric

- Instructions: Juice all the ingredients together. Beetroot is known for its ability to improve blood flow and stamina, making it perfect for an energy boost. Turmeric adds anti-inflammatory benefits, while carrots and apples provide sweetness and vitamins.

Ingredients That Promote Vitality

Certain ingredients are particularly effective at promoting vitality and sustaining energy levels throughout the day:

- Beetroot: Rich in nitrates, beetroot enhances blood flow, improving oxygen delivery to muscles and the brain. This results in increased stamina and mental clarity.

- Spinach: High in iron, spinach supports the production of red blood cells, which carry oxygen throughout the body, helping to prevent fatigue.

- Ginger: Ginger stimulates digestion and circulation, aiding in energy production and helping to maintain steady energy levels.

- Citrus Fruits: Oranges, lemons, and grapefruits are high in vitamin C, which is essential for the production of energy at the cellular level. They also help to refresh and hydrate the body.

Detox and Cleansing

Detoxifying Juice Recipes

Detoxification is the process of removing toxins from the body, and juicing can play a crucial role in this process. The right juices can support liver function, aid digestion, and help flush out harmful substances. Here are some detoxifying juice recipes:

1. Green Detox Elixir

- Ingredients: 1 cucumber, 1 handful of kale, 1 green apple, 1 lemon, 1-inch piece of ginger

- Instructions: Juice all the ingredients together. This juice is loaded with chlorophyll, which helps cleanse the liver and kidneys, while ginger supports digestion and reduces inflammation.

2. Citrus Cleanse

- Ingredients: 2 oranges, 1 grapefruit, 1 lemon, 1-inch piece of turmeric

- Instructions: Juice all the ingredients together. The high vitamin C content in this juice supports the body's natural detoxification processes and helps neutralize free radicals.

3. Carrot and Apple Detox

- Ingredients: 3 carrots, 2 apples, 1-inch piece of ginger, 1 lemon

- Instructions: Juice all the ingredients together. Carrots and apples are high in fiber and antioxidants, which help to cleanse the digestive tract and eliminate toxins.

Benefits of a Juice Cleanse

A juice cleanse involves consuming only fresh vegetable and fruit juices for a period of time, usually ranging from one to three days. The purpose of a juice cleanse is to give your digestive system a break while flooding your body with nutrients. Benefits of a juice cleanse include:

- Enhanced Detoxification: A juice cleanse supports the liver and kidneys in removing toxins from the body, helping to purify the blood and improve overall health.

- Improved Digestion: By consuming only liquids, a juice cleanse gives the digestive system a rest, allowing it to reset and heal.

- Increased Nutrient Intake: Juice cleanses provide a concentrated source of vitamins, minerals, and antioxidants, helping to boost the immune system and protect against disease.

- Mental Clarity: Many people report feeling more focused and clear-headed during and after a juice cleanse, as the body’s energy isn’t diverted to digestion.

Weight Loss and Management

Juices to Support Weight Loss

Juicing can be an effective tool for weight loss when incorporated into a balanced diet. The key is to choose ingredients that are low in calories but high in nutrients, helping you feel full and satisfied without overeating. Here are some weight-loss-friendly juice recipes:

1. Slimming Green Juice

- Ingredients: 1 cucumber, 2 celery stalks, 1 handful of spinach, 1 green apple, 1 lemon

- Instructions: Juice all the ingredients together. This juice is low in calories but high in fiber, which helps to keep you full. The lemon also helps to boost metabolism.

2. Berry Blast

- Ingredients: 1 cup of mixed berries (blueberries, strawberries, raspberries), 1 apple, 1 handful of spinach

- Instructions: Juice all the ingredients together. Berries are low in calories and high in antioxidants, making this juice a great option for weight management.

3. Carrot and Ginger Metabolism Booster

- Ingredients: 3 carrots, 1 apple, 1-inch piece of ginger

- Instructions: Juice all the ingredients together. Carrots are rich in fiber, and ginger helps to boost metabolism, making this juice a great addition to a weight loss plan.

Tips for Incorporating Juicing into a Weight Loss Plan

- Replace High-Calorie Snacks: Swap out high-calorie snacks for a nutrient-dense juice to reduce overall calorie intake while still feeling satisfied.

- Use Juices as Meal Supplements: While juices shouldn't replace meals entirely, they can be used as supplements to add extra nutrients and keep you full between meals.

- Choose Low-Sugar Ingredients: Opt for vegetables and low-sugar fruits like berries, cucumbers, and leafy greens to keep your juice low in calories and sugar.

- Stay Hydrated: Drinking plenty of water in addition to your juices is essential for weight loss and overall health. It helps to keep you full and flushes out toxins.

Immune Boosting

Immune-Boosting Ingredients

Your immune system is your body's first line of defense against illness, and certain ingredients can help strengthen it. Incorporating immune-boosting ingredients into your juices can provide a natural way to protect your health. Here are some key ingredients to include:

-Citrus Fruits: Oranges, lemons, and grapefruits are high in vitamin C, which is crucial for immune function.

-Ginger: Ginger has powerful anti-inflammatory and antimicrobial properties that help to fight off infections.

- Turmeric: Turmeric contains curcumin, a compound with strong anti-inflammatory and antioxidant effects that can boost immunity.

- Garlic: While not common in juices, garlic can be added in small amounts for its potent immune-boosting properties. It’s known for its ability to fight bacteria and viruses.

Recipes to Strengthen the Immune System

1. Citrus Immunity Booster

- Ingredients: 2 oranges, 1 lemon, 1 grapefruit, 1-inch piece of ginger

- Instructions: Juice all the ingredients together. This juice is loaded with vitamin C and antioxidants to help strengthen the immune system.

2. Golden Immunity Juice

- Ingredients: 1 orange, 1 carrot, 1-inch piece of turmeric, 1-inch piece of ginger

- Instructions: Juice all the ingredients together. Turmeric and ginger add anti-inflammatory and immune-boosting benefits, while the orange and carrot provide a sweet, nourishing base.

3. Green Immunity Elixir

- Ingredients: 1 cucumber, 1 handful of spinach, 1 green apple, 1 lemon, 1-inch piece of ginger

- Instructions: Juice all the ingredients together. This juice is packed with vitamins, minerals, and antioxidants to support overall immune health.

Juicing offers a versatile and delicious way to support various health goals, from boosting energy and detoxifying the body to aiding in weight loss and strengthening the immune system. By selecting the right ingredients and recipes, you can tailor your juicing routine to meet your specific needs and enjoy the numerous benefits that come with it. In the next chapter, we'll explore how to create your own juice recipes, allowing you to customize your juicing experience even further.

Chapter Five

Juicing for Specific Health Conditions

In the journey to better health, juicing stands as a versatile and potent tool, tailored to address specific health conditions. By selecting the right combination of fruits, vegetables, and herbs, you can create juices that not only taste delightful but also target particular areas of your health. In this chapter, we'll explore how juicing can support heart health, improve digestion, enhance skin health, and boost mental wellness. Let's delve into these health-focused juices and the ingredients that make them powerful allies in your health journey.

Heart Health

Your heart is the powerhouse of your body, tirelessly pumping blood to keep you alive. It's crucial to nourish it with the right nutrients. Juicing for heart health involves incorporating ingredients known for their cardiovascular benefits, such as those rich in antioxidants, fiber, and healthy fats.

Ingredients that Promote Cardiovascular Health:

- Beets: High in nitrates, beets help dilate blood vessels, reducing blood pressure and improving circulation.
- Pomegranates: Rich in antioxidants like punicalagins and anthocyanins, pomegranates reduce oxidative stress and lower cholesterol levels.
- Leafy Greens (Spinach, Kale): These are high in dietary nitrates, potassium, and magnesium, which help regulate blood pressure.
- Berries (Blueberries, Strawberries): Packed with anthocyanins, berries help reduce blood pressure and improve arterial function.
- Flaxseeds: A great source of omega-3 fatty acids and fiber, flaxseeds help lower cholesterol and inflammation.

Heart-Healthy Juice Recipes:

1. Beetroot & Berry Boost:

- 1 beetroot
- 1 cup blueberries
- 1 cup spinach
- 1 apple
- 1 tablespoon flaxseed (optional, ground)

- Juice everything and stir in the ground flaxseed for a heart-healthy kick.

2. Pomegranate Power:

- 1 cup pomegranate seeds
- 1 orange
- 1 handful kale
- 1 teaspoon honey (optional)
- Juice and enjoy a sweet, tangy drink packed with heart benefits.

Digestive Health

A well-functioning digestive system is key to overall health. Juices designed to improve digestion can help alleviate bloating, promote gut health, and soothe the digestive tract. The focus here is on ingredients that provide fiber, probiotics, and anti-inflammatory properties.

Ingredients that Soothe the Digestive System:

- Ginger: Known for its anti-inflammatory and stomach-soothing properties, ginger helps reduce nausea and improve digestion.
- Pineapple: Contains bromelain, an enzyme that aids in breaking down proteins and improving digestion.
- Cucumber: Hydrating and gentle on the stomach, cucumber helps flush out toxins and reduce bloating.
- Papaya: Rich in papain, a digestive enzyme, papaya aids in breaking down food and improving nutrient absorption.

- Aloe Vera:Contains compounds that soothe the digestive tract and promote healthy bowel movements.

Juices to Improve Digestion:

1. Ginger-Pineapple Digestive Aid:
   - 1 cup pineapple
   - 1 inch ginger root
   - 1 cucumber
   - 1 apple (for sweetness)
   - Juice and enjoy this refreshing, digestion-friendly drink.

2. Papaya Cooler:
   - 1 cup papaya
   - 1/2 cucumber
   - 1/2 lemon
   - 1 tablespoon aloe vera gel (from the leaf)
   - Juice and savor the cooling, stomach-soothing properties of this blend.

Skin Health

Healthy, glowing skin often reflects a well-nourished body. Juices packed with vitamins, antioxidants, and hydrating ingredients can do wonders for your skin. The goal here is to boost collagen production, reduce inflammation, and hydrate from within.

Ingredients that Promote Healthy Skin:

-Carrots: High in beta-carotene, which the body converts into vitamin A, essential for skin health.

- Cucumber: Provides hydration and is rich in silica, which helps maintain skin elasticity.
- Oranges: Rich in vitamin C, crucial for collagen production and skin repair.
- Aloe Vera: Soothes the skin and provides hydration from the inside out.

- Turmeric: Known for its anti-inflammatory and antioxidant properties, turmeric helps reduce redness and combat free radicals.

Juices for Glowing Skin:

1. Radiant Skin Elixir:
   - 2 carrots
   - 1 cucumber
   - 1 orange
   - 1 inch turmeric root
   - Juice all ingredients for a vibrant, skin-loving beverage.

2. Citrus Glow:
   - 1 orange
   - 1 grapefruit
   - 1/2 cucumber
   - 1 tablespoon aloe vera gel (from the leaf)
   - Juice and bask in the glow of this citrusy, hydrating drink.

Mental Health and Wellness

Mental health is just as important as physical health, and the right juice can help boost mood, improve mental clarity, and support overall brain health. The focus here is on ingredients that reduce inflammation, provide essential fatty acids, and support neurotransmitter function.

Ingredients that Support Brain Health:

- Blueberries: Rich in antioxidants and phytonutrients that protect the brain and improve cognitive function.
- Walnuts: High in omega-3 fatty acids, walnuts support brain health and improve mood.
- Spinach:Contains folate, which helps produce neurotransmitters that regulate mood.
- Bananas: Rich in tryptophan, a precursor to serotonin, which helps regulate mood.

- Turmeric: Its active compound, curcumin, has been shown to enhance mood and cognitive function.

Juices to Boost Mood and Mental Clarity:

1. Brain Power Juice:
   - 1 cup blueberries
   - 1 handful spinach
   - 1 banana
   - 1 tablespoon walnut oil (optional)
   - Juice and enjoy a mental clarity-boosting drink.

2. Golden Mind Refresher:
   - 1 orange
   - 1 inch turmeric root
   - 1 apple
   - 1/2 lemon
   - Juice for a refreshing, mood-enhancing beverage.

Juicing offers a simple, effective way to target specific health conditions with the power of nature's best ingredients. By incorporating these recipes into your routine, you can support your heart, improve digestion, enhance skin health, and boost mental wellness—one delicious sip at a time.

Chapter Six

Integrating Juicing into Your Lifestyle

Juicing is a powerful way to enhance your health, but like any new habit, it requires consistency and integration into your daily life to reap its full benefits. This chapter will guide you through making juicing a regular part of your routine, even with a busy schedule. We'll explore portable juicing solutions for those on the go and discuss how to combine juicing with other healthy practices to create a holistic approach to wellness.

Daily Juicing Habits

The key to long-term success with juicing lies in turning it into a daily habit. Incorporating fresh juice into your day doesn't have to be time-consuming or complicated. With a bit of planning and some helpful tips, you can easily make juicing a natural part of your routine.

How to Make Juicing a Daily Habit:

1. Start Small and Build Consistency:

Begin by setting a realistic goal, such as having one juice a day. Choose a time that fits naturally into your routine, whether it's a morning boost, an afternoon pick-me-up, or an evening refreshment.

As you become more comfortable, you can gradually increase the variety of your juices.

2. Prepare in Advance:

Planning is crucial to maintaining a daily juicing habit. Set aside time once or twice a week to wash, peel, and chop your ingredients. Store them in airtight containers in the fridge, so they're ready to go when you need them. This small step can save you a lot of time during busy mornings.

3. Create a Routine:

Link your juicing habit to an existing part of your routine, such as your morning coffee or post-workout snack. This will help establish a strong connection between juicing and another daily activity, making it easier to stick with.

Time-Saving Tips for Busy Schedules:

1. Use a High-Quality Juicer:

Invest in a juicer that is efficient and easy to clean. Slow or masticating juicers are ideal for retaining nutrients, but they can be more time-consuming to clean. Centrifugal juicers are faster but may not extract as much juice. Find a balance that works for your lifestyle.

2. Make Juice in Batches:

If you know you'll have a busy week, consider making a large batch of juice and storing it in the fridge. While fresh juice is best consumed immediately, many juices can be stored in airtight containers for up to 48 hours without significant nutrient loss.

3. Consider Pre-Made Juices:

On particularly hectic days, having a few pre-made, cold-pressed juices on hand can help you stick to your juicing habit. Look for brands that prioritize organic, fresh ingredients with no added sugars or preservatives.

Juicing on the Go

Life can be unpredictable, but your juicing routine doesn't have to suffer when you're on the move. With the right tools and a little creativity, you can enjoy the benefits of juicing wherever you are.

Portable Juicing Solutions:

1. Invest in a Portable Blender:

Portable blenders are compact, battery-powered devices that allow you to make fresh juice or smoothies anywhere. These are perfect for travel, work, or even outdoor activities. Simply pack your pre-cut ingredients and blend when you're ready to enjoy your juice.

2. Juice Packs and Frozen Cubes:

Prepare juice packs by freezing portions of juice in ice cube trays or small containers. When you're ready to enjoy your juice, simply blend or shake the frozen cubes with water or coconut water. This is an excellent way to have fresh juice on hand without the need for a juicer.

3. Reusable Bottles and Jars:

Invest in high-quality, reusable bottles or jars that keep your juice fresh and are easy to carry. Look for bottles made of glass or BPA-free plastic to ensure your juice stays as pure as possible. These are ideal for taking your juice to work, the gym, or on trips.

Tips for Maintaining Your Juicing Routine While Traveling:

1. Research Local Options:

When traveling, research local juice bars or cafes that offer fresh, cold-pressed juices. This can be a convenient way to keep up with your juicing habit without the need to carry equipment.

2. Pack Your Essentials:

If you're staying somewhere with kitchen facilities, consider packing a small juicer or portable blender. You can also bring along a supply of non-perishable juicing ingredients like citrus fruits, ginger, and beetroot powder.

3. Plan Ahead:

Before your trip, prepare a list of ingredients that travel well and are easy to find at local markets. This can include apples, carrots, celery, and lemons. Planning ahead will make it easier to continue your juicing routine, even when you're away from home.

Combining Juicing with Other Healthy Practices

Juicing is a fantastic way to boost your health, but its benefits are amplified when combined with other wellness practices. By taking a holistic approach to your health, you can create a well-rounded lifestyle that supports your overall well-being.

Complementary Wellness Practices:

1. Mindful Eating:

Alongside juicing, adopt a mindful eating practice. Focus on whole, unprocessed foods, and pay attention to your hunger and fullness cues. This will help you maintain a balanced diet and avoid the temptation to rely solely on juice for nutrition.

2. Regular Exercise:

Combine your juicing routine with regular physical activity. Whether it's yoga, walking, or strength training, exercise supports detoxification, boosts energy levels, and enhances mental clarity. Post-workout juices rich in antioxidants and electrolytes can aid in recovery.

3. Hydration:

While juice can contribute to your daily fluid intake, it's important to drink plenty of water throughout the day. Staying hydrated helps maintain your energy levels, supports digestion, and keeps your skin glowing.

Holistic Approach to Health and Wellness:

1. Stress Management:

Incorporate stress management techniques such as meditation, deep breathing, or journaling into your routine. Juicing can be a part of your self-care regimen, with certain ingredients like ashwagandha, lemon balm, or chamomile helping to reduce stress.

2. Sleep Hygiene:

Prioritize good sleep hygiene by maintaining a regular sleep schedule and creating a relaxing bedtime routine. Consider including calming juices, like those made with tart cherries or lavender, which can promote better sleep.

3. Community and Support:

Surround yourself with a supportive community of like-minded individuals who share your health goals. Whether it's a local juicing group, an online community, or friends who enjoy healthy living, having support can motivate you to stick to your healthy lifestyle.

Integrating juicing into your lifestyle doesn't have to be daunting. By establishing daily habits, finding portable solutions, and combining juicing with other healthy practices, you can create a sustainable and holistic approach to health and wellness. This chapter is your guide to making juicing a natural, enjoyable, and effective part of your everyday life.

Chapter Seven

Overcoming Challenges and Common Mistakes

Juicing offers a multitude of health benefits, from increased energy levels to better skin health. However, like any new endeavor, it comes with its own set of challenges and potential pitfalls. In this chapter, we'll explore common juicing issues and provide practical solutions for overcoming them. Additionally, we'll delve into strategies for staying motivated on your juicing journey, sharing success stories and testimonials to inspire you.

Troubleshooting Common Juicing Issues

Starting a juicing routine can be exciting, but it's not uncommon to encounter some hurdles along the way. Whether it's dealing with bitter flavors or finding that your yield isn't as high as expected, these challenges can be frustrating. Here's how to troubleshoot some of the most common juicing issues.

Bitter or Unpleasant Tastes:

One of the most frequent complaints among new juicers is the occasional bitter or unpleasant taste. This can be off-putting, especially if you're expecting a refreshing and sweet drink.

1. Balance Flavors:

Bitter tastes often arise from using too many leafy greens or vegetables like kale, spinach, or celery, which are highly nutritious but can overpower your juice. To balance the flavor, add naturally sweet ingredients like apples, carrots, or oranges. A small piece of ginger or a squeeze of lemon can also brighten the flavor and reduce bitterness.

2. Use Fresh Ingredients:

The freshness of your ingredients plays a crucial role in the taste of your juice. Overripe or wilted produce can lead to a less-than-pleasant flavor. Always use fresh, crisp fruits and vegetables, and try to juice them as soon as possible after purchase.

3. Experiment with Ratios:

If your juice is too bitter, experiment with the ratios of ingredients. Start with a base of fruits or vegetables you enjoy and gradually add in smaller amounts of stronger-tasting greens. Over time, your palate may adjust, allowing you to incorporate more nutrient-dense but bitter greens.

4. Strain Your Juice:

Sometimes, the bitterness can come from small bits of pulp or seeds left in the juice. Straining your juice through a fine mesh sieve or cheesecloth can remove these particles, resulting in a smoother, more pleasant taste.

Low Yield and Efficiency:

Another common issue is not getting as much juice from your produce as you expected. This can be disappointing, especially if you've invested in high-quality ingredients.

1. Choose the Right Juicer:

The type of juicer you use significantly impacts your yield. Masticating (slow) juicers tend to extract more juice from leafy greens and fibrous vegetables than centrifugal juicers. If you find that your yield is consistently low, it might be worth investing in a higher-quality juicer that's designed for efficiency.

2. Prep Your Produce:

Proper preparation can make a big difference in juice yield. For example, chopping fibrous vegetables like celery into smaller pieces before juicing can help break down the fibers and increase yield. Similarly, peeling citrus fruits or cutting off tough skins can prevent clogging and improve efficiency.

3. Juice in the Right Order:

To maximize yield, juice softer, high-water-content fruits like cucumbers or oranges first. This helps lubricate the juicer for tougher ingredients like leafy greens or carrots. If your juicer has a reverse function, use it occasionally to unclog the machine and push through any remaining pulp.

4. Re-Juice the Pulp:

After your first round of juicing, check the pulp. If it's still quite wet, you can run it through the juicer again to extract more juice. Some people also find creative uses for pulp in recipes like soups, muffins, or veggie patties, ensuring that nothing goes to waste.

Staying Motivated

Maintaining motivation is essential for long-term success with juicing. While the initial enthusiasm can carry you through the first few weeks, it's common for motivation to wane over time. Here are some tips to help you stay committed and inspired on your juicing journey.

Tips for Staying Committed to Juicing:

1. Set Clear Goals:

Whether your goal is to boost your energy, improve your skin, or support weight loss, having a clear purpose can keep you motivated. Write down your goals and refer to them regularly to remind yourself why you started juicing in the first place.

2. Track Your Progress:

Keeping a journal of your juicing journey can be incredibly motivating. Record the recipes you try, note how you feel after drinking your juice, and track any improvements in your health. Seeing your progress in black and white can encourage you to keep going.

3. Create a Routine:

Incorporate juicing into your daily routine by linking it to another habit, such as your morning workout or afternoon break. Making juicing a non-negotiable part of your day will help you stay consistent, even when life gets busy.

4. Get Creative with Recipes:

Boredom can quickly derail your juicing efforts. To keep things interesting, experiment with new ingredients and flavor combinations. Try adding herbs like mint or basil, or explore seasonal produce for variety. Keeping your palate excited will make juicing something you look forward to.

5. Join a Community:

Connecting with others who are also on a juicing journey can provide a strong support system. Join online forums, social media groups, or local juicing meetups to share tips, recipes, and experiences. The sense of community can be a powerful motivator.

Success Stories and Testimonials:

Hearing about the experiences of others can be incredibly inspiring and help reinforce your commitment to juicing. Below are a few testimonials from individuals who have transformed their health through consistent juicing.

1. Sarah's Story:

Sarah, a busy mother of two, struggled with low energy and frequent colds. After incorporating daily green juices into her routine, she noticed a significant boost in her energy levels and rarely fell ill. "Juicing has been a game-changer for me," Sarah shares. "I never thought I could feel this good just by adding a daily juice."

2. John's Journey:

John, a 45-year-old professional, was looking for a natural way to manage his high blood pressure. He started juicing beets, celery, and other heart-healthy vegetables every morning. Over time, his blood pressure stabilized, and he no longer needed medication. “Juicing didn’t just improve my health; it gave me my life back,” John says.

3. Emily’s Experience:

Emily, a college student, was dealing with persistent acne and dull skin. After researching the benefits of juicing, she began drinking a juice rich in carrots, oranges, and turmeric daily. Within a few months, her skin cleared up, and she regained her confidence. “My skin has never looked better,” Emily beams. “Juicing is now a permanent part of my beauty routine.”

4. Michael’s Transformation:

Michael, a retiree, wanted to lose weight and improve his overall health. He replaced one meal a day with a nutrient-dense juice and gradually adopted a more balanced diet. Over the course of a year, he lost 30 pounds and felt more energetic than he had in decades. “Juicing was the jumpstart I needed,” Michael reflects. “It helped me change my lifestyle for the better.”

These success stories highlight the transformative power of juicing when combined with consistency and a positive mindset. Whether you’re dealing with a specific health issue or simply looking to enhance your well-being, juicing can be a valuable tool on your journey.

Overcoming challenges and avoiding common mistakes is an essential part of any successful juicing journey. By addressing issues like bitter flavors and low yield, you can ensure that your juicing experience remains enjoyable and effective. Staying motivated is equally important, and with the right strategies and inspiration, you can make juicing a lifelong habit that supports your health and wellness goals. Remember, every challenge you overcome brings you one step closer to the vibrant health you desire.

Chapter Eight

Advanced Juicing Techniques

Juicing is more than just a way to enjoy fresh fruits and vegetables; it's a powerful tool for enhancing your health and well-being. Once you've mastered the basics, you may find yourself eager to explore more advanced juicing techniques. This chapter will delve into two exciting aspects of advanced juicing: juice fasting and detox programs, and creating your own custom juice recipes. By the end of this chapter, you'll be equipped to take your juicing journey to the next level.

Juice Fasting and Detox Programs

Benefits and Considerations:

Juice fasting, also known as juice cleansing, is a practice where you consume only juice for a set period, typically ranging from one to seven days. The idea behind juice fasting is to give your digestive system a break while flooding your body with nutrients from fresh fruits and vegetables. Proponents of juice fasting claim that it can help detoxify the body, improve digestion, boost energy levels, and promote weight loss.

1. Detoxification:

The human body is exposed to various toxins through food, water, and the environment. While the liver and kidneys naturally detoxify the body, juice fasting is believed to support these organs by reducing the intake of processed foods, sugars, and unhealthy fats, allowing the body to focus on eliminating toxins.

2. Increased Nutrient Intake:

Juice fasting allows you to consume a large quantity of fruits and vegetables in a condensed form. This high concentration of vitamins, minerals, and antioxidants can help strengthen your immune system, improve skin health, and support overall well-being.

3. Digestive Rest:

A juice fast gives your digestive system a break from processing solid foods, which can help reduce bloating and improve gut health. Some people report feeling lighter and more energized during and after a juice fast.

4. Mental Clarity:

Many who have tried juice fasting report enhanced mental clarity and focus. This could be due to the elimination of processed foods and sugars from the diet, which can cause fluctuations in blood sugar levels and energy.

How to Safely Conduct a Juice Fast:

While juice fasting can offer numerous benefits, it's important to approach it with caution, especially if you're new to fasting or have underlying health conditions. Here's how to conduct a juice fast safely.

1. Consult a Healthcare Professional:

Before starting a juice fast, especially if you have any health conditions or are on medication, it's crucial to consult with a healthcare professional. They can help you determine if juice fasting is appropriate for you and provide guidance on how to proceed safely.

2. Start Slow:

If you're new to juice fasting, start with a short fast, such as a one-day or three-day cleanse. This allows your body to adjust to the change and helps you gauge how you feel during the fast. You can gradually increase the duration of your fasts as you become more experienced.

3. Choose the Right Juices:

During a juice fast, it's important to consume a variety of juices that provide a balance of nutrients. Focus on juices made from a mix of fruits and vegetables to ensure you're getting a wide range of vitamins and minerals. Avoid juices that are too high in sugar, as they can cause spikes in blood sugar levels.

4. Stay Hydrated:

In addition to drinking juice, make sure you're consuming plenty of water throughout the day. This helps support detoxification and keeps you hydrated. Herbal teas and coconut water can also be included to provide variety.

5. Listen to Your Body:

Pay attention to how your body feels during the fast. It's normal to experience some mild symptoms, such as headaches or fatigue, as your body adjusts. However, if you feel excessively weak, dizzy, or unwell, it's important to break the fast and consult a healthcare professional.

6. Ease Back into Solid Foods:

Once your juice fast is complete, don't rush back into eating solid foods. Start with light, easily digestible foods, such as fruits, vegetables, and soups, before gradually reintroducing more complex meals. This helps your digestive system transition smoothly back to normal eating.

Creating Your Own Recipes

Balancing Flavors and Nutrients:

Creating your own juice recipes is one of the most rewarding aspects of juicing. Not only does it allow you to tailor the flavors to your preferences, but it also gives you control over the nutritional content. Here's how to balance flavors and nutrients when crafting your custom juices:

1. Understand Flavor Profiles:

When creating a juice recipe, it's important to understand the different flavor profiles of the ingredients you're using. Fruits and vegetables can be sweet, tangy, bitter, or earthy. Balancing these flavors is key to creating a juice that is both delicious and nutritious.

- Sweet: Apples, carrots, beets, and pineapples add natural sweetness to your juice. These ingredients are great for masking the bitter or earthy flavors of leafy greens and other vegetables.

- Tangy:Citrus fruits like lemons, limes, and oranges provide a tangy kick that can brighten up your juice. A small amount of ginger can also add a spicy tang.

- Bitter: Kale, spinach, and dandelion greens are known for their bitter taste. While these ingredients are incredibly healthy, it's best to pair them with sweeter fruits or vegetables to balance the bitterness.

- Earthy: Root vegetables like beets and carrots have an earthy flavor that pairs well with both sweet and tangy ingredients.

2. Focus on Nutrient Density:

When creating a juice, aim for a combination of ingredients that provide a broad spectrum of nutrients. Include a variety of fruits and vegetables to ensure you're getting a mix of vitamins, minerals, and antioxidants. For example, pairing vitamin C-rich oranges with iron-rich spinach can enhance iron absorption in the body.

3. Incorporate Superfoods:

Superfoods are nutrient-dense ingredients that can boost the health benefits of your juice. Consider adding a handful of spinach or kale for a dose of vitamins A and K, or a scoop of spirulina for added protein and antioxidants. Other superfoods like turmeric, chia seeds, and flaxseed can also be incorporated for additional benefits.

4. Experiment with Herbs and Spices:

Fresh herbs and spices can elevate the flavor of your juice while providing additional health benefits. Mint, basil, and cilantro add freshness, while ginger and turmeric offer anti-inflammatory properties. Don't be afraid to experiment with small amounts of these ingredients to discover new and exciting flavor combinations.

Tips for Experimenting with New Ingredients:

Juicing is a creative process, and experimenting with new ingredients can lead to delicious discoveries. Here are some tips for exploring new ingredients in your juice recipes:

1. Start Small:

When trying a new ingredient, start with a small amount. This allows you to gauge the flavor and ensure it doesn't overpower the juice. You can always add more if needed.

2. Mix Familiar with Unfamiliar:

Pairing a new or unfamiliar ingredient with something you already enjoy can make it easier to adjust to the new flavor. For example, if you're trying kale for the first time, mix it with the sweetness of apples and carrots.

3. Research Health Benefits:

Learning about the health benefits of different fruits and vegetables can inspire you to try new combinations. For example, if you're interested in improving digestion, you might experiment with ingredients like fennel, ginger, or papaya.

4. Keep a Recipe Journal:

As you experiment with new ingredients and combinations, keep a journal of your recipes. Note the quantities, flavor profile, and how you felt after drinking the juice. This will help you refine your recipes over time and create a personalized collection of favorites.

5. Don't Be Afraid of Failure:

Not every juice you create will be a masterpiece, and that's okay. Part of the fun of juicing is the experimentation process. If a recipe doesn't turn out the way you hoped, make adjustments and try again. Over time, you'll develop a better understanding of what works and what doesn't.

Advanced juicing techniques like juice fasting and creating your own recipes offer exciting opportunities to enhance your health and take your juicing practice to the next level. By understanding the benefits and considerations of juice fasting, you can safely incorporate this practice into your wellness routine. Meanwhile, experimenting with new ingredients and balancing flavors will allow you to craft delicious, nutrient-dense juices that are tailored to your unique tastes and health goals. As you continue your juicing journey, remember that the possibilities are endless, and every glass of juice is a step toward a healthier, more vibrant life.

The Journey to Better Health

As we reach the end of this book, it's important to reflect on the journey we've embarked upon together. Juicing is more than just a trend or a passing health fad—it's a powerful tool for transforming your health and well-being from the inside out. Whether you're a seasoned juicer or just starting out, the principles and techniques we've explored can serve as a lasting foundation for a healthier, more vibrant life.

Recap of Key Points:

Throughout this book, we've delved into the many aspects of juicing, from the basics to more advanced techniques. We've discussed the importance of incorporating fresh fruits and vegetables into your daily routine and explored the specific health benefits that juicing can offer. From promoting heart health and improving digestion to enhancing skin radiance and boosting mental clarity, juicing has the potential to positively impact nearly every aspect of your well-being.

We also looked at practical tips for integrating juicing into your lifestyle, making it a sustainable habit rather than a short-term fix. By establishing daily juicing habits, finding portable solutions for juicing on the go, and combining juicing with other healthy practices, you're well on your way to creating a holistic approach to health.

Moreover, we've tackled some of the common challenges and mistakes that can arise on your juicing journey, providing solutions and encouragement to help you stay motivated. Whether you're dealing with bitter tastes, low yield, or simply struggling to stay committed, the tools and strategies shared in this book are designed to keep you on track.

Finally, we ventured into advanced juicing techniques, exploring the benefits of juice fasting and detox programs, and offering guidance on creating your own custom juice recipes. These advanced techniques open up a world of possibilities, allowing you to tailor your juicing practice to your specific health goals and personal preferences.

Encouragement to Continue the Juicing Journey:

The journey to better health is ongoing, and juicing is a valuable companion along the way. As you continue to explore the world of juicing, remember that it's not about perfection but progress. Each glass of juice is a step toward nourishing your body, revitalizing your spirit, and embracing a healthier lifestyle.

There will be days when you feel like you've mastered the art of juicing and days when it feels like a challenge. On those challenging days, remind yourself of why you started this journey in the first place. Reflect on the positive changes you've experienced—whether it's more energy, clearer skin, or a greater sense of well-being. Let these small victories fuel your motivation to keep going.

Don't be afraid to experiment and explore new ingredients, flavors, and techniques. The beauty of juicing lies in its versatility and adaptability. Whether you're looking to cleanse, energize, or simply enjoy a delicious and nutritious drink, there's juice out there for you.

As you move forward, consider sharing your juicing journey with others. Inspire friends and family to join you, exchange recipes, and celebrate the benefits of this vibrant practice together. Community support can be a powerful motivator, and spreading the joy of juicing can have a ripple effect, contributing to a healthier, happier world.

In conclusion, juicing is more than just a dietary choice—it's a lifestyle, a commitment to your health, and a celebration of the nourishing power of nature. So, raise your glass to the journey ahead, and remember that with each sip, you're investing in a healthier, more vibrant version of yourself. Here's to your continued success on the journey to better health!

Appendices

The following appendices are designed to serve as a comprehensive reference guide to support your juicing journey. Whether you're looking to deepen your understanding of the nutritional value of ingredients, plan your juicing around seasonal produce, clarify terminology, or explore additional resources, this section has you covered.

Nutritional Information of Common Juicing Ingredients

Understanding the nutritional content of the fruits and vegetables you use in your juices is crucial for maximizing the health benefits of your juicing practice. Below is a list of common juicing ingredients along with their key nutrients and health benefits:

- Kale

  - Nutrients: Vitamin K, Vitamin A, Vitamin C, Calcium, Iron

  -Benefits: Supports bone health, boosts immunity, promotes healthy skin

- Spinach

  - Nutrients: Vitamin K, Folate, Iron, Magnesium

  - Benefits: Aids in blood clotting, supports muscle and nerve function, enhances red blood cell production

- Carrots

  - Nutrients: Beta-carotene, Vitamin A, Potassium, Fiber

  - Benefits: Improves eye health, supports heart health, promotes digestive health

- Beets
  - Nutrients: Folate, Manganese, Potassium, Nitrates
  - Benefits: Lowers blood pressure, boosts stamina, supports liver detoxification
- Ginger
  - Nutrients: Gingerol, Vitamin C, Magnesium, Potassium
  - Benefits: Reduces inflammation, aids digestion, boosts immunity
- Apples
  - Nutrients: Vitamin C, Fiber, Potassium
  - Benefits: Supports heart health, promotes digestive health, provides antioxidant protection

- Celery

  - Nutrients: Vitamin K, Folate, Potassium, Fiber

  - Benefits: Reduces inflammation, supports digestive health, promotes hydration

- Cucumbers

  - Nutrients: Vitamin K, Vitamin C, Potassium, Silica

  - Benefits: Hydrates the body, supports skin health, aids in detoxification

- Oranges

  - Nutrients: Vitamin C, Folate, Potassium, Fiber

  - Benefits: Boosts immunity, promotes heart health, supports skin health

- Pineapple

  - Nutrients: Vitamin C, Bromelain, Manganese

  - Benefits: Aids digestion, reduces inflammation, supports immune function

This is just a glimpse of the nutrient-rich ingredients you can incorporate into your juices. By understanding the nutritional profiles of these foods, you can create balanced and healthful juices tailored to your specific needs.

Seasonal Produce Chart

Juicing with seasonal produce not only ensures fresher, more flavorful ingredients but also supports local farmers and is often more cost-effective. Below is a general guide to what produce is in season during different times of the year. Keep in mind that availability may vary depending on your location.

- Spring

  - Vegetables: Asparagus, Spinach, Radishes, Kale

  - Fruits: Strawberries, Pineapple, Mango, Kiwi

- Summer

  - Vegetables: Zucchini, Cucumber, Bell Peppers, Tomatoes

  - Fruits: Watermelon, Blueberries, Peaches, Plums

- Fall

  - Vegetables: Beets, Carrots, Sweet Potatoes, Squash

  -Fruits: Apples, Pears, Grapes, Pomegranates

- Winter

- Vegetables: Kale, Brussels Sprouts, Leeks, Cabbage

- Fruits: Oranges, Grapefruits, Persimmons, Cranberries

Juicing with the seasons allows you to take advantage of peak freshness and nutrient content. It also adds variety to your juicing regimen, helping you enjoy a broader range of flavors and benefits.

Glossary of Terms

Understanding specific terms and concepts is essential as you delve deeper into the world of juicing. Below is a glossary of common juicing-related terms to help you navigate your journey with confidence:

- Cold-Pressed Juice: Juice extracted using a hydraulic press, which minimizes heat and oxidation, preserving nutrients and enzymes.

- Centrifugal Juicer: A juicing machine that uses a fast-spinning blade to extract juice from produce, typically more affordable but may result in nutrient loss due to heat.

- Masticating Juicer: A slow-speed juicer that "chews" the produce to extract juice, retaining more nutrients and producing higher-quality juice.

- Enzyme: Proteins that catalyze chemical reactions in the body, including those involved in digestion and metabolism.

- Antioxidant: Compounds that protect cells from damage caused by free radicals, reducing the risk of chronic diseases.

- Detoxification: The process of removing toxins from the body, often supported by consuming nutrient-dense juices.

-Nutrient Density: The concentration of essential nutrients in a food relative to its calorie content, with higher nutrient density foods offering more vitamins and minerals per calorie.

-Oxidation: A chemical reaction that can lead to the degradation of nutrients in juice, often minimized by cold-pressing.

Resources and Further Reading

To continue expanding your knowledge and refining your juicing practices, here are some recommended resources for further reading:

- Books:

  - The Juice Fasting Bible by Sandra Cabot, M.D.

  - Juice It to Lose It by Joe Cross

  - The Reboot with Joe Juice Diet by Joe Cross

  - The Big Book of Juices by Natalie Savona

- Websites:

  - [Juicing for Health](https://www.juicing-for-health.com): A comprehensive site with articles, recipes, and tips on juicing for various health conditions.

  - [Reboot with Joe](https://www.rebootwithjoe.com): A resource hub for juice fasting, recipes, and community support.

  - [Juice Recipes](https://www.juicerecipes.com): An extensive collection of juicing recipes categorized by health benefits.

- Apps:

  -Juice Master by Jason Vale: Offers hundreds of recipes, along with shopping lists and expert advice.

  - Juice Recipes (iOS/Android): Features an array of juice recipes and nutritional information.

This appendices section is intended to be a valuable resource you can return to time and again as you refine your juicing skills and continue your journey to better health. With the right knowledge, tools, and resources at your fingertips, you're well-equipped to make juicing a lasting and impactful part of your wellness routine.

About the Author

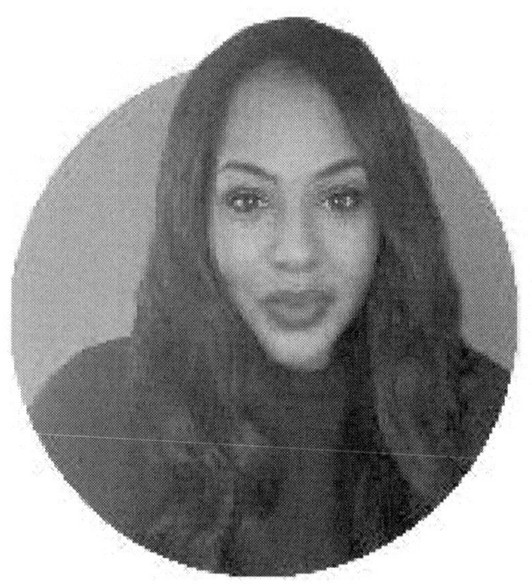

Dr. Monique Rodgers is an international bestselling author, CEO, visionary, master business coach, certified vegan health coach, motivational speaker, entrepreneur, educator, and literary genius. Dr. Rodgers excels today as a notable writing coach, founder, and serial entrepreneur. Throughout the course of her career, she has written such prolific works such as Hello! My name is Millennial. Picking up the Pieces, The Mystical Land of Twinville, Falling in Love with Jesus, Accelerate, Overcoming Writer's Block, Just Breathe, Called to Intercede Volumes 1-14 and I am Black History and many more. She has also been included as a co-author in collaborations such as Jumpstart Your Mind, Speak Up We Deserve to be Heard, Finding Joy in the Journey Volume 2, and Let the Kingdompreneurs Speak. Due to her outstanding breadth of experience, Dr. Rodgers has been featured on Rachel Speaks radio program, The Love Walk Podcast, The Glory Network, God's Glory Radio Show, The Miracle Zone, The Healing Zone, The Joyce Kiwani Adams Show, Coach Monique Ph.D. radio show, and many more. She has graced numerous platforms worldwide. She served as a TV host for WATCTV. She has been featured in Heart and Soul magazine, My Story the Magazine, and Kish Magazine's Top 20 Authors of 2021. She has also been featured in Marquis Who's Who in America 2021-2022. She also assisted in various volunteer work including an executive team member for Lady Deliverers Arise, Aniyah Space, and a board member for the I Am My Sister organization. She is also a certified master business coach, certified vegan health coach, and a health advocate. She has served in various leadership positions in business and in ministry. She is currently an Awakening Prayer hub leader for the city of Raleigh under the tutelage of Apostle Jennifer LeClaire. She is an ambassador for Kingdom Sniper Institute under the mentorship of Evangelist Latrice Ryan. As an expert in her field, Dr. Rodgers earned an undergraduate degree through Oral Roberts University as well as a Master of Science degree and a doctorate in global leadership through Colorado Technical University. She has also studied at The Black Business School online. Looking towards her future, Dr. Rodgers intends to expand upon her expertise and continue serving through ministry for God. She aspires to help over one hundred authors to complete and publish their books, help intercessors to draw closer to God and help train marketplace prophets and leaders for success.

To stay connected with Dr. Monique Rodgers

Contact information:
www.getwriteoncoaching.com
www.meetdrmonique.com
Facebook: www.facebook.com/moniquerodgers2
Instagram: @drroyalty7
Twitter: @DrMonique7
LinkedIn: Dr. Monique Rodgers
YouTube: Dr. Monique Rodgers
Clubhouse: @DrMonique7
Email: calledtointerecede@gmail.com

Made in the USA
Middletown, DE
23 December 2024